Powerful Life

How to Cultivate Energy, Vitality, and Focus

Table of Contents

The energy of the mind is the essence of life.

Chapter 1. Introduction

Unveiling the power within you is now within reach thanks to our Special Report titled "Powerful Life: How to Cultify Energy, Vitality, and Focus." This illuminating guide is not only a boon for those yearning for a more vibrant way of living, but also those who have been seeking ways to channel their inner strength and focus in a world that often leaves us drained and directionless. Unlike complicated technical manuals, this is a joyous exploration of practical and powerful strategies we could all use to bring more energy, vitality, and focus into our daily lives. Trust us, by the time you reach the end of this introductory paragraph, you'd be more than excited to delve deeper into the bountiful resource that this Special Report is. Feel the surge of a whole new wave of energy and vitality just waiting to be unlocked - and it's all just a page away!

Chapter 2. Unlocking Your Inner Powerhouse: Introduction

Our fascination and curiosity with human potential have been longstanding. Over time, the premise of understanding the intricacies of human capability, unlocking deeper layers of strength, and deciphering the codes to personal energy and focus have heightened significantly. This chapter dwells on these cornerstones of human potential, taking you on a journey that swings wide the doors to your inner powerhouse, enabling you to adopt a lifestyle that emanates with energy, vibrancy, and focus.

2.1. The Essence of Personal Power

Personal power is the ability to control the environment around you. This power can arise from various factors such as knowledge, experience, or interpersonal abilities. But at its core, personal power is about harnessing and directing your internal energy, waking up to your innate potential, and turning them into action. It's about fearlessly navigating life and its challenges whilst staying true to your authentic self. Once you kick-start the engine of your personal power, no obstacle will be too large, no dream too far-fetched.

2.2. Energy, Vitality, and Focus: The Three Pillars

Energy, vitality, and focus are three pillars that sustain our personal power. Energy is the fundamental force driving our every action and thought. Vitality, on the other hand, is not just about the physical state of being strong but also a steady state of energetic enthusiasm and robustness in all elements of life. Focus, the third pillar, is the ability to concentrate one's energy and attention in the direction of a chosen goal or task.

Each individual possesses these three vital elements, but the extent to which they are tapped into, harnessed, and manipulated can vary significantly, and therein lies the difference between those who merely survive and those who truly thrive.

2.3. The Potential Within: Unbounded and Awaiting Discovery

The latent power within us is a treasure trove waiting to be discovered. Often, it's unbounded and untapped, residing quietly under layers of fear, uncertainty, and social conditioning. Unlocking this power involves acknowledging its existence, unearthing it and embracing it despite the fear of the unknown, and finally, channeling it towards growth, success, and well-being.

2.4. Nurturing the Seeds of Innate Power

While each one of us is born with seeds of power, they need to be nurtured and cared for to sprout and grow. This nurturing process entails fostering positive mindsets, instilling healthy habits, surrounding oneself with energy amplifiers, and continually fueling our drive to learn and grow. When these seeds get the requisite nurturing, the sprouts solidify into the bedrock of personal power, steering us towards the manifestation of a fulfilling life.

2.5. Demystifying the Process of Unlocking

One of the first steps in the process of unlocking your power is understanding yourself, your desires, strengths, limitations, and abilities. It is about acknowledging and embracing the entirety of your being, including the darker or weaker parts, and working on building your personal power around this comprehensive version of yourself. This process requires the right guidance, tools, and eventually, a practical, achievable plan.

Never consider the process of unlocking your personal powerhouse a sprint. It is a gradual process, a marathon that wants you to stay patient, consistent, and resilient. Each day you choose to embrace and harness your innate power is a step forward, a step closer towards a life brimming with energy, vitality, and focus. Thus, embark on this journey, not with the aim to reach an unrealistic overnight transformation, but with the intention to progressively grow and evolve each day.

Remember, the process of unlocking is not about becoming someone new, but uncovering the real you. It's about investigating ourselves, our potentials, capabilities, frailties, aspirations, and deepest fears. It's about shining a light into dark corners and finding, there, in the dust, the power and abilities that have lying dormant, waiting for you to breathe life into them. So, let's put on our explorer's hat and embark on this thrilling expedition toward self-discovery and self-empowerment.

2.6. Embracing the Journey: A Life of Energy, Vitality, and Focus

In this chapter, we have scratched the surface of personal power and set the stage for the journey towards a life infused with greater energy, vitality, and focus. The subsequent chapters in this book will delve deeper into the various strategies, practices, and pathways that can lead you to unlock your inherent power, allowing you to lead a life of purpose, passion, and potential.

Your journey to tapping into your inner powerhouse and attaining a grander life awaits, and this is only the beginning. Keep turning the pages, and let's commence on this exciting journey together.

With this, we conclude our introduction, aiming at preparing you for the forthcoming detailed exploration. You can anticipate a comprehensive, applicable guide crafted to assist you in understanding and tapping into your inherent energy reservoir. It is now time to stride onto the path of self-discovery and empowerment, time to power up the engine of your life.

Chapter 3. Vitalize: Full Spectrum Health for Greater Energy

In our quest to lead a potent life brimming with energy, vitality, and focus, the first stop is nurturing a full spectrum of health. This envisions a holistic approach, treating our body as a complete system rather than fractured parts. We will traverse the several components of our physical constitution, mental well-being, and spiritual alignment that propels us toward a healthy and energy-filled existence.

3.1. Basics of Full Spectrum Health

The term 'Full Spectrum Health' embodies the totality of health and wellness. It isn't confined to physical well-being alone but extends to mental, emotional, and spiritual wellness. This mindset treats the body as a synergistically operating system where the health of one component impacts the others. Energy and vitality are not standalone aspects but an outcome of total health care.

3.2. Nutrition: The Cornerstone of Health

The power of proper nutrition, the fuel that drives our bodies, can never be overstated. If we are what we eat, then consuming energy-dense and nutrient-rich food will invariably lead to a healthier, more energetic self. The age-old wisdom of balancing our diet with fruits, vegetables, whole grains, lean meats, and avoiding processed food, trans fats holds true under any health paradigm.

Similarly, staying hydrated is crucial. Dehydration can cause fatigue and limit cognitive functions. Aim to drink at least eight glasses of water a day or more if engaged in strenuous physical activities or if you dwell in a hot climate.

3.3. Exercise: Energize Your Body

Engaging with regular physical activity is a sure-fire way to ramp up your energy reserves. Besides strength and aerobic workouts, incorporate activities that increase flexibility and promote balance. Creating a well-rounded exercise regimen can yield dividends in the form of energy and vitality.

One such example includes combining strength training workouts with yoga or Pilates. While the former can build muscle and improve metabolism, the latter can work wonders for flexibility and mindfulness, fostering a harmonious balance.

3.4. Sleep: The Silent Healer

Getting an adequate amount of quality sleep is non-negotiable for full-spectrum health. Insufficient sleep can cause an energy slump and deteriorate overall health. Most adults require around seven to nine hours of sleep each night.

Focus on improving sleep hygiene, which comprises maintaining regular sleep hours, creating a restful sleep environment, and avoiding activities that might hamper sleep close to bedtime.

3.5. Mental health: The Invisible Pillar

Mental health feeds into our energy reserves in more ways than one. Chronic stress, anxiety, and depression can lead to fatigue and sap us of our vitality. Engage in activities that foster mental wellness such as mindfulness, meditation, and recreational hobbies.

A healthy social life and maintaining positive relationships contribute significantly to mental well-being. Invest time and effort in nurturing relationships that create joy and offer support.

3.6. Spiritual Alignment: Energy from Within

Lastly, spiritual health often gets overlooked, yet plays a significant role. Inner peace and contentment contribute to our overall vitality, manifesting as an energy source from within. Activities such as meditation, time spent in nature, practicing gratitude, and following a purpose greater than oneself serve to enhance spiritual health.

Integrating all these facets together creates a powerful symphony that resonates with energy, vitality, and focus. A well-rounded approach to health becomes the cornerstone to amplify these qualities in our life. By adopting strategies outlined in this chapter, you embark on an immersive journey toward a fuller, more vibrant life that is charged with energy and teeming with vitality.

Chapter 4. Profound Impact: Changing Your Diet, Changing Your Energy

The evidence is mounting and cannot be ignored: the food we consume has a significant impact on our energy levels, mood, productivity, and overall health. Buckle up as we journey down the entrancing avenue of dietary changes for an energetic transformation.

4.1. The Power of Nutrition

Just as a car runs smoothly on high-quality fuel, our bodies thrive on a superior nutritional diet. The profound impact of nutrition on energy begins with understanding the basics. Carbohydrates, proteins, and fats are the essential macro-nutrients that directly translate into energy. However, the quality, quantity, and timing of these macro-nutrients greatly influence how we feel and function.

Carbohydrates are the body's primary source of energy, quickly converted into glucose for immediate use or stored as glycogen for later needs. Proteins and fats provide a slower, more sustained release of energy. Consuming a balanced mix of these macros ensures a steady, lasting stream of vitality throughout the day.

4.2. The Role of Micro-nutrients

Micro-nutrients, despite being necessary in much smaller quantities, also play crucial roles in energy metabolism. Vitamins and minerals such as B vitamins, iron, magnesium, and iodine help convert food into fuel, regulate metabolism, repair cellular damage, and contribute to the production of energy-transporting molecules in our bodies.

Micro-nutrient deficiencies can lead to fatigue, diminished stamina, and decreased focus. Therefore, incorporating a diverse range of fruits, vegetables, grains, lean meats, and other natural, nutrient-dense foods into your diet is essential.

4.3. Nutrient Timing and Energy

The timing of when we ingest nutrients, known as nutrient timing, impacts our energy levels and our overall health. Distributing nutrients evenly across meals and snacks throughout the day can prevent energy slumps and overeating, while allowing efficient metabolic processing.

Indeed, skipping meals or indulging in high sugar and processed food can cause substantial fluctuations in your blood sugar levels, leading to erratic energy peaks and troughs. Maintaining steady blood sugar levels by having smaller, regular meals and snacks can help sustain your energy and keep your focus sharp all day long.

4.4. The Hydration Element

Water makes up about 60 percent of our bodies and is involved in virtually every bodily process. Even slight dehydration can cause fatigue and decreased cognitive function. Staying adequately hydrated ensures proper brain function and body temperature regulation, both vital for maintaining energy.

4.5. The Confluence of Diet, Exercise, and Rest

While diet is undeniably a critical component of our energy, vitality, and focus, it's one part of a broader triad. Integrating a balanced diet with regular physical activity and sufficient rest creates a synergetic effect that amplifies each component's contribution to energy creation and sustainability.

4.6. Final Thoughts and Practical Tips

A healthier diet isn't about a complete overnight transformation but incorporating gradual changes. For instance, swapping white bread for whole grain bread, introducing more fruits and vegetables into your meals, reducing processed foods, ensuring a regular intake of lean proteins and complex carbohydrates, and staying well-hydrated can make a remarkable difference.

Remember, your diet is your fuel. Through understanding and acting upon the profound connection between diet and energy, you can set yourself on the path toward a life of vibrancy, clarity, and prosperity.

Change is often challenging, but the reward of enhanced vitality and focus is well worth the hurdles. Your journey towards a balanced life of sustained energy now begins with that single step. Empower yourself with the gift of optimal nutrition and witness the transformative effects on your energy and life. Be patient, be diligent, but most of all, be open to reaping the profound rewards this chapter promises. It's time for a dietary revolution, a switch to real foods and wholesome habits that promise a lifetime of energy, vitalizing your body, mind, and spirit for the extraordinary journey of life.

Chapter 5. Mindfulness: Simple Practices for Improved Focus

Mindfulness, a practice dating back thousands of years, has recently resurfaced with newfound significance in the face of a fast-paced, distracted world. The concept is beguilingly simple: stay present, remain in the moment, and recenter your focus. Yet, to truly harness the benefits of this practice isn't an easy feat in today's world. To bridge the gap, this chapter peels away the layers of mindfulness, proposing simplistic yet profoundly influential exercises that can pivot us towards an enriched life of amplified focus, equanimity, and energy.

5.1. Embracing the Concept of Mindfulness

Mindfulness translates to being totally present, being fully aware of where we are and what we're doing, and not overly reacting or feeling overwhelmed by what's happening around us. Despite common misconceptions, mindfulness is not about eradicating all thoughts or achieving a state of ceaseless tranquility. Instead, it promotes a keen awareness of our thoughts, feelings, and sensations in real-time, without judgment or the urge to react impulsively.

5.2. The Benefits of Mindful Practice

Numerous research studies have documented the transformative powers of mindfulness. These benefits span enhanced concentration, improved mental clarity, reduced anxiety, and better emotional resilience. By honing an individual's capacity to focus on what's going on in the moment, we beneficially rewire the brain, making it easier to zero in on tasks and regulate emotional responses.

5.3. Mindfulness Techniques to Enhance Focus

With benefits made abundantly clear, let's uncover some elementary yet effective mindfulness techniques to help you build unprecedented focus and mental clarity.

5.4. Focus on the Breath

The simplest, most foundational mindfulness practice centers on observing the breath. You can follow this practice in a quiet space, free from distractions:

1. Take a comfortable seated posture.

2. Close your eyes gently.

3. Direct your attention to your breathing.

4. Now, simply observe your breath. How does it feel going in? How about going out?

5. If you notice your attention wandering (and it will), simply redirect it back to the breath.

5.5. Body Scan

This meditative practice encourages an intimate understanding of our physical presence:

1. Lie down in a relaxing position. Close your eyes.

2. Focus on different sections of your body, starting from the toes and gradually moving upwards towards your head.

3. Observe any sensations or discomforts without attempting to alter them.

4. At each part, you might choose to silently name the body part and acknowledge the sensation you have in that part.

5.6. Walking Meditation

This practice is best for those who find tranquility in motion:

1. Choose the location, ideally somewhere quiet and serene.

2. Begin to walk at a natural pace.

3. Pay attention to your steps, observing the sensations that occur with the lifting and descending of each foot.

4. Be conscious of your breathing and the sensation of the wind against your skin.

5.7. Eating Mindfully

This practice infuses mindfulness into a daily activity - eating:

1. At your next meal, take a moment to appreciate the appearance and aroma of your food.

2. With each bite, chew slowly, savoring every flavor and texture.

3. Try to keep your focus on the food and the act of eating, rather than letting your mind wander elsewhere.

5.8. Meditation: The Mind's Gym

Meditation, a formal expression of mindfulness, is similar to the exercise of muscles. Regular sessions help us build mental strength, fostering a habit of sustained focus. Initiating a daily practice, even if just for five minutes a day, can create a significant shift in your ability to handle distractions and maintain attention.

5.9. Dealing with Distractions

Distractions, internal or external, are inevitable when practicing mindfulness. But they are not the enemy. The key to managing them is accepting their existence and choosing to gently redirect our attention back to the chosen focus point. Ingeniously, distractions provide an opportunity to strengthen our concentration muscles each time we return our focus.

5.10. Incorporating Mindfulness into Daily Life

Successfully applying mindfulness does not just occur in dedicated periods of meditation. You can seamlessly integrate mindfulness into your daily activities - a practice commonly termed as 'informal mindfulness'. This might involve immersing in the sensations while washing dishes, listening attentively during a conversation, or absorbing the variegated sights during a neighborhood walk.

The journey into mindfulness, like venturing into any novel terrain, might seem intimidating. However, making small iterative changes, and indulging in these simple practices consistently, can lead you towards triumphant outcomes over time. So, get started, stay patient, and let mindfulness be your beacon to an improved focus, signaling the dawn of a more energized, vibrant life.

Chapter 6. Optimize Sleep: Sleeping Your Way to Increased Vitality

The science of sleep has been the focus of rigorous research for decades, given its pivotal role in our overall well-being. This chapter aims to provide in-depth insights and strategies about optimizing sleep patterns for enhanced vitality and productivity.

6.1. Principle of Sleep

The first essential understanding is the principle behind sleep. Yes, we all require sleep, but comprehending why could contribute significantly to improving your arsenal of self-optimizing tools. Sleep principally serves as a restorative process for the body and mind. During sleep, the body regenerates cells, repairs tissue, synthesizes proteins, and allows your brain to organize and process information from the day.

Sleep is characterized by different stages, primarily classified into two categories: Rapid Eye Movement (REM) and Non-Rapid Eye Movement (NREM), each having unique and essential roles in rejuvenation and restoration. It's not only the number of hours spent sleeping but also the quality and progression through these stages that influence our vitality.

6.2. Creating an Ideal Sleep Environment

The environment you create for your sleep is crucial. It would be best to consider factors like lighting, temperature, and noise, all of which significantly impact your sleep quality.

Blinds or curtains can help achieve a dark room, and earplugs can be considered in case of unavoidable noise. Keep the room temperature modestly cool, around 60-67 degrees Fahrenheit. This temperature range is generally considered optimal for good sleep for most individuals.

6.3. The Role of Diet in Sleep Optimization

What you ingest plays a significant role in defining your sleep pattern. Consuming caffeine or alcohol close to bedtime can hinder your sleep cycle and prevent you from entering the deeper, more restful stages of sleep. Choose to consume cherries, walnuts, kiwi, or warm milk, which contain nutrients that can naturally boost your melatonin levels, enhancing your sleep quality.

6.4. Routinizing Sleep

Respect your circadian rhythm - the body's internal clock managing sleep-awake cycles over a 24-hour period. Going to bed and waking up at consistent times will help regulate your body's clock and could help you fall asleep and stay asleep for the night. Good habits like avoiding electronic gadgets, doing light exercises, and reading a book before bedtime could help calm the mind, aiding in an improved sleep cycle.

6.5. Sleep and Physical Activity

Engage in regular physical activity. Studies show a strong link between regular exercise and improved sleep. Regular physical activity can help you fall asleep faster and enjoy deeper sleep, thereby increasing your energy levels.

6.6. The Power of Napping

Consider incorporating power naps into your routine. Research shows that a short nap of 20-30 minutes can help to improve mood, alertness, and performance without leaving you feeling groggy or interfering with nighttime sleep. But remember to keep it limited; excessive napping could lead to sleep problems.

6.7. Mindfulness for Better Sleep

Practicing mindfulness and relaxation techniques can be an effective strategy to combat sleep troubles. Techniques like controlled breathing, progressive muscle relaxation, and visualization can help you unwind, leading to a more peaceful transition into sleep.

6.8. Sleep Disorders: Recognize and Seek Help

If despite trying all these tactics you still struggle with sleep, then it might be an indication of a sleep disorder. Recognizing this is crucial. Insomnia, sleep apnea, restless legs syndrome- these are just a few examples of conditions that could be hampering your sleep. The message here is not to self-diagnose but to seek professional help if you continually struggle with quality sleep.

Optimizing sleep is not about chasing an eight-hour rule that might not fit all. It is more about understanding and catering to your body's unique needs, forming habits that support rather than interfere with your sleep, and treating sleep as a critical component of your path to increased vitality and focus. Embrace the suggestions that resonate with you, and experience your life's energy transform subtly but surely.

Chapter 7. Movement Magic: Harnessing Physical Activity for More Energy

Let's start our journey towards energy harnessing by understanding that physical activity isn't simply a means towards weight loss or muscle building—it's a gateway to a world of enhanced vitality and elated energy levels. Many individuals overlook this dimension of physical movement, paying undue attention to aesthetic outcomes, while the true power underlying their act of exercising remains unexplored. Now, step by step, we shall unfold the magic engulfed within physical movement and how you, too, can reap its benefits.

7.1. Understanding the Energy-Movement Connection

In the most basic terms, our body converts the food we eat into energy. This energy is then used to power every movement—big, small, visible, or internal. Regular physical activity increases our body's efficiency in this energy conversion process, leading to better energy management and improved vitality. But just how does this occur?

Delving deeper, every cell in our body contains mitochondria referred to as the 'powerhouses' of the cell. Regular physical exertion leads to an increase in both the size and number of these mitochondria, hence boosting our body's capacity to produce energy. Over time, this enhanced energy production inculcates a feeling of enhanced vigor and vitality within individuals who adopt regular movement routines.

Additionally, regular physical activity promotes better blood circulation, ensuring well-oxygenated and well-nourished cells—another catalyst that boosts energy levels within the body.

7.2. Identifying the Best Movement Practices for Energy Enhancement

Every individual has a unique body and hence, the 'best' physical activity that optimizes one's energy frequency varies. However, certain practices hold unanimous benefits.

Start by trying modest activities such as brisk walking or cycling that gradually help uplift your energy levels. They are also less likely to lead to energy crashes post-workout, hence offering a sustainable approach to energy management.

Resistance and weight training, although slightly more intense, also prove beneficial in increasing muscle mass which in turn, aids in boosting your basal metabolic rate and energy creation.

Don't forget to incorporate flexibility routines and mind-body practices like yoga and tai chi. These forms of movement aid in maintaining the optimal functioning of your bodily systems, reduce stress, and tend to have great benefits for overall vitality.

7.3. Creating an Effective Movement Routine

The aim here isn't to transform you into a marathon runner or an Olympic weightlifter overnight; instead, the focus lays on cultivating a habit of regular physical movement. To make this happen, let's devise a sustainable routine.

Decide on a minimum duration every day that you can commit to for exercise—15 minutes, half an hour, or more. Ensure you exercise at least 3-5 days a week, and spread your activity throughout the day if necessary.

Make your routine enjoyable! Include activities you love that also fall under physical exertion, like dancing or hiking. This will make you look forward to your movement session each day as opposed to dreading it.

Don't forget to warm up before workouts to prepare your body for movement and cool down posts to help it relax. Skipping these steps can lead to quick exhaustion and injury.

7.4. The Role of Recovery: Many a Times Overlooked Aspect of Energy Creation

Remember, our body isn't a machine. It requires relaxation and rejuvenation to continue functioning effectively. Therefore, after periods of physical exertion, ensure that you provide sufficient time for your body to recover.

Sleep is a natural recovery mechanism. Make sure you're getting enough sleep every night to allow your body to repair and get ready for the next day.

Recovery also includes taking care of your gut. Introduce protein-rich foods in your diet after a workout session to facilitate quicker recovery.

Hope this comprehensive guide helps you harness your potential energy through a prudent movement routine. Remember, the path to elevated vitality through movement isn't a sprint, it's more of a marathon. Be patient with yourself and enjoy the journey!

Chapter 8. Ditch the Drain: Identifying and Managing Energy Vampires

In myriad ways, the world surrounds us with invisible yet pervasive forces that can detrimentally drain our vitality. These forces, colloquially known as "energy vampires," can exist in many forms. They lurk in our relationships, our environment, even within our minds. They have the capacity to suck the zest out of life, leaving us feeling drained and devoid of the vigor necessary for a fulfilling and productive existence.

8.1. Identifying Energy Vampires

Awareness is the initial step in combatting these draining forces. Everything around us exerts an influence. From people and their words, workplace environments, to our homes, events, news, situations, even thoughts can be sources of energy drain. These entities feed on our energy, giving us very little, if anything, in return, thereby becoming energy vampires. Being able to correctly and swiftly identify these powerful siphons is crucial to maintaining one's energy levels.

Let's now delve deeper into these draining forces, with specific examples and the impact they exert on us.

8.1.1. People

Certain individuals in our lives, often called Narcissists or Egocentrics can unconsciously(or consciously) drain your energy. Interactions with them leave you feeling tired, emotionally depleted, and negative. They often demand much attention, assert superiority, or impose their problems on others relentlessly.

8.1.2. Environments

Workplaces, schools, and even homes can sometimes turn into energy-draining zones. Massively competitive or hostile workplaces, stressful academic environments, cluttered, and disharmonious homes often sap our vital energy.

8.1.3. Events and Situations

Highly demanding events like nonstop meetings, chronic crisis occurrences, or any situations riddled with conflict and disarray can seriously drain us.

8.1.4. News and Social Media

Continuous exposure to negative news or being persistently active on social media also has a substantial draining impact.

8.1.5. Thoughts and Emotions

Our own thoughts and emotions can serve as energy vampires. Negative thinking, perpetual anxiety, and unrelenting stress ensure a constant drain on your energy reserves.

8.2. Handling Energy Vampires

Once you've identified the vampires, managing them becomes the next crucial step. The process involves conscious decision-making, foresight, and specific strategies to prevent energy dissipation.

8.2.1. Establishing Boundaries

A surefire way to manage energy vampires is by setting strong boundaries. This applies predominantly to relationships that tend to drain you. Say 'no' when necessary, assert your personal space and time, making it less accessible for the energy vampires.

8.2.2. Optimizing Environments

Arrange your environments to promote rather than drain energy. For a workplace or home, ensure it's well organized, sufficiently lit, and comfortable. A harmonious environment ensures a net gain rather than a loss in energy.

8.2.3. Mindfulness and Conscious Consumption

Whether it's about dealing with situations, news, or social media, mindfulness comes to your aid. Be aware of what you consume, mentally and emotionally. Limit exposure to stress-inducing situations, negative news, and mindless social media scrolling.

8.2.4. Positive Thinking and Emotional Regulation

Cultivating a positive mindset and learning to regulate our emotions can hugely help in managing the energy drain. Meditation, practicing gratitude, or cognitive-behavioral techniques may be useful in achieving this.

8.3. Sustaining Energy Levels

Safeguarding one's energy levels is not a one-time task. It must become a part of one's lifestyle. Like a diligent gardener, we must prune away the overgrowth that strangles our vitality, while nurturing those aspects that enliven and energize us.

Remember, ensuring that the sources of energy drain have been suitably handled is not enough. Make it a point to review and reassess. Our environments, interactions, and challenges may change over time, necessitating adjustment of your strategies accordingly.

By constant awareness and vigilant management, it becomes possible to effectively identify and manage these energy vampires. Your reward will be a more vibrant and more fulfilling life. One in which you dictate the flow of your energy rather than it being subjected to invisible external drains. As you continue your journey through this life of power, remember that you hold the reins. These energy management strategies can allow you to take charge, turning the tables on the energy vampires once and for all.

Chapter 9. Powerful Routines: Designing Your Day for Maximum Focus

To materialize the tangible and intangible benefits of maximum focus, one must understand the paramount importance of well-designed daily routines. This chapter will take you on a detailed exploration of how to design your day for a laser-sharp focus.

9.1. Understanding the Role of Routines

Quite frequently we overlook the role of routines in shaping our productivity and focus. Routine provides a sense of structure, eliminating the need for constant decision making and reducing anxiety over what needs to be done next. As a result, routines can free up our mental bandwidth and allow us to focus more on tasks that require our full attention and creative input. By cultivating powerfully designed routines, we facilitate a mental environment that is conducive for achieving maximum focus and, subsequently, peak productivity.

9.2. Crafting Your Morning Routine: A Strong Start

A well-orchestrated morning routine serves as a formidable foundation for a day brimming with energy and focus. To design such a routine, consider integrating activities that invigorate your body, stimulate your mind, and nurture your spirit. For your body; consider practices like stretching, yoga, or a brisk walk to get your blood circulating. For your mind; activities such as reading, writing, or studying could prove beneficial. Lastly, for your spirit; meditative practices such as deep breathing, visualization, or peaceful solitude can induce a calm state of mind.

9.3. Attuning Your Midday Routine: Keeping the Momentum

As the day progresses, staying focused can start to feel like an uphill battle. Thus, a well-designed midday routine is crucial for maintaining your momentum and revitalizing your focus. Begin by scheduling regular breaks; research has shown that taking short breaks after every 50-90 minutes of work can substantially improve focus. During these breaks, engage in activities that are polar opposites of your work: if you've been working on a computer, take a stroll outside; if your work is physically demanding, relax and read a calming book. Moreover, consider strategic meal timings as untimely meals can disrupt your flow.

9.4. Honing Your Evening Routine: Ensuring Quality Rest

The importance of an evening routine is often underestimated. A skilfully crafted evening routine does not only ensure an effective close to your day but also sets you up for success the next day. Prioritize relaxation and disconnect from technological devices at least one hour before sleep. This prevents the disruption of your natural sleep cycle caused by blue light emitted from screens. Engage in calming activities such as reading a book, meditating, or gentle stretching. Preparing for the next day could also be beneficial; laying out clothing, planning meals, and jotting down next day's to-do list can save time & mental energy.

9.5. Evaluating and Adjusting Your Routine

As with any endeavor, honest self-reflection is key for success. Regularly evaluate your routine to ensure it still aligns with your goals and is promoting optimal focus. Allow room for flexibility and tweaks. As you grow and evolve, so should your routines. Experiment with different activities, timings, and variables to find what best suits your lifestyle.

A well-structured routine doesn't merely provide a roadmap for the day; it also fosters the conditions necessary for achieving a laser-sharp focus, an indispensable tool in our pursuit of personal and professional success. Whether it's honing your morning ritual or tweaking your evening schedule, it's the little details that make a world of difference in cultivating focus. Step back, evaluate, adjust, and remain fluid - this is the key to creating a powerful routine that paves the way for the best version of you.

Chapter 10. A Balanced Life: Establishing Harmony in Body, Mind, and Work

Life is a delicate dance of various components, where imbalance in one can touch off a domino effect, causing upheaval across the whole. To truly harvest all the energy, vitality, and focus within us, it is crucial to establish harmony in three principal realms - body, mind, and work. This involves learning to attune to our inherent rhythms, streamlining our daily chores, aligning our work with our passions, fostering rich relationships, and nurturing our inner being. As we explore these intricate realms and how they overlap, you may find insights that lead you to a renewed sense of balance and a deeper understanding of your innate power.

10.1. Navigating the Vessel: The Body

The cornerstone of our existence, the physical body, is the vessel that enables us to interact with the world. Providing it with the proper care is vital to preserving its functionality. A well-nourished, adequately rested, and regularly exercised body optimizes the available energy for focus, creativity, and productivity.

When thinking about nourishing your body, consider both what you consume and when you consume it. Nutrient-rich, natural foods provide the essential building blocks for physical health and vitality. Human bodies thrive on regular, predictable meal times, aiding metabolism and digestive health.

Rest is another non-negotiable facet of physical health. The advent of artificial lighting and digital devices has disrupted natural sleep patterns for many, negatively impacting both energy levels and focus. Taking steps to ensure regular, high-quality sleep is paramount in restoring vitality.

Physical activity, such as regular exercise, contributes significantly to our energy levels, improving sleep, mood, and overall bodily functions. From brisk walking to high-intensity interval training, incorporating movement into your day can have significant effects on your wellness.

10.2. The Interior Universe: The Mind

While the body is our tangible realm, our minds deal with the intangible. A mind filled with incessant thoughts, worries, or regrets can drain energy and inhibit focus. By developing habits to declutter your mind, you can increase mental clarity, reduce stress, and amplify your focus.

An effective way to find peace of mind is to commune with nature. It could be a walk in the woods, watching a sunset, or tending to a garden. Nature has a calming effect on the mind. It brings us back to the present and awakens our senses.

Meditation is another powerful tool to quiet the mind. It allows you to observe your thoughts without getting entangled in them. Regular meditation can reduce stress, increase attention span, and promote emotional health. Even a few minutes of daily meditation can result in noticeable improvements.

10.3. Energy in Action: Work

Work is where our body and mind converge to create value. It is here that our energy, when focused, allows us to produce, contribute, and make a difference. Optimizing our work environment and aligning our tasks with our passions can lead to a significant uptick in both productivity and satisfaction.

An orderly workspace reduces distractions and promotes efficient workflow. Investing time in task management strategies—like the Eisenhower box or the Pomodoro technique—can help in organizing your workload and prioritizing tasks.

It's equally essential to ensure that your work aligns with your passions and values. Work that you love, that challenges you and fulfills you, will naturally engage your focus and enhance your vitality. Conversely, work that drains you or feels misaligned with your character can deplete your energy.

10.4. The Confluence: Body, Mind, and Work

Harmony is achieved when body, mind, and work are in sync, allowing unhindered flow of energy. The practices and techniques detailed above can support you in nurturing and maintaining this balance.

Regular check-ins with yourself can help to identify areas of imbalance, providing opportunities to make adjustments before adverse effects arise. This could mean altering your diet, incorporating a new mindfulness technique, or changing a part of your work routine.

The journey towards a balanced life involves continual learning, adapting, and refining based on your unique needs and circumstances. It may involve trial and error, and require patience and self-compassion. But in the end, the reward is a life of amplified energy, sharpened focus, and sustained vitality. Find your balance, and unleash your true potential.

Chapter 11. Sustaining Vitality: Creating a Long Lasting Life of Energy and Focus

Imagine standing at the edge of a vast lake, the water surface so calm it's near-perfect mirror reflects the picturesque sky. Toss a pebble in the serene water, and watch as the single ripple starts to form, disrupting the calm. It starts small but gradually expands outward until it emanates across the entire surface of the lake. This ripple effect, in essence, can be likened to the concept of vitality, energy and focus that we are targeting. Each positive action towards sustaining these aspects in your life starts small, yet with the potential to create massive, encompassing effects. Don't disregard the power of those tiny daily habits, as they hold the key to creating a long-lasting life of energy and focus.

11.1. The Drift towards Lifestyle Change: Not a Revolution But an Evolution

Creating and, more importantly, sustaining vitality requires a shift in our everyday behaviors. However, we don't advocate for sudden, drastic lifestyle changes; such revamps often demand too much effort upfront and might discourage you from pursuing true, sustainable change. Instead, consider the subtle art of evolving your lifestyle habits - easy and consistent changes that build upon each other to bring about profound impact.

11.2. The Four Pillars of Vitality: Nutrition, Movement, Restoration, and Mindset

To build a life pulsating with high vitality, we propose a comprehensive approach addressing four main areas: Nutrition, Movement, Restoration, and Mindset.

Nutrition: Food is our primary energy source, and the quality of energy we derive significantly depends on the quality of sustenance we ingest.

Movement: Regular physical activity vitalizes your body, promotes mental clarity, and allows efficient circulation of energy within.

Restoration: Sufficient rest and proper sleep give your mind and body the time to rejuvenate and recover from daily rigors.

Mindset: A positive and clear mind attracts energy and focuses like nothing else.

11.3. Plate of Power: How Nutrition Sustains Energy and Focus

Considering nutrition first, cultivating a balanced diet is critical for sustained vitality and focus. Emphasize whole foods that are rich in complex carbohydrates, lean proteins, and healthy fats. These nutrients are the building blocks of enduring energy. Furthermore, hydration plays an integral role in maintaining optimal body functions, so don't forget to incorporate adequate fluid intake.

11.4. Motion is Potion: The Role of Physical Activity

Next, movement is a celebration of what your body can do and is fundamental for sustaining energy. Incorporate varied physical activities into your routine, from vigorous workouts to gentle stretches. Remember, the goal is not solely about physical intensity but consistent movement that energizes you and keeps your momentum high.

11.5. Recharge to Reemerge: The Importance of Rest and Sleep

Restoration, the third pillar, underscores the importance of rest and sleep. As essential as punchy workouts and being active is, you must give your body a proper chance to recover and rejuvenate. Establish sound sleep hygiene and recognize when your body is pleading for some downtime.

11.6. Powerful Mindset: The Nexus of Energy and Focus

Finally, the power of mindset. No guide to vitality can be comprehensive without addressing the efficiency of maintaining a positive mental scenery. Mental strategies like meditation, mindfulness, and cognitive reframing can help you harness the power of positivity, paving the way for sustained vitality and focus.

11.7. Ripples into Waves: Making Small Changes that Compound

Transforming these identified pillars into a lifestyle that perpetuates vitality and focus requires small but mighty changes. From mindful eating to establishing an exercise plan that you love, from setting sleep schedules to routinely practicing mindfulness, these tiny teardrop actions can compound to create a profound ripple that transforms into an encompassing wave of ongoing vitality and focus.

Remember, sustainable change does not come from short-term stints but rather a long-term commitment to evolving your lifestyle habits. The power to revitalize your life and focus better lies within you—and the small, seemingly insignificant changes you introduce to your everyday life.

As our exploration of "Sustaining Vitality: Creating a Long-Lasting Life of Energy and Focus" concludes, remember that each day offers a fresh canvas, waiting to be painted with vitality-filled colors. Cultivate these habits steadily, measure your progress, and give yourself permission to evolve. The ripple will soon turn into the wave of energy and focus you seek. In this sea, you will find the power to understand, direct, and sustain your vitality like a never-ending rhythmic dance, syncing beautifully with your life's melody.